1 MONTH OF
FREE
READING

at

www.ForgottenBooks.com

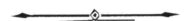

By purchasing this book you are eligible for one month membership to ForgottenBooks.com, giving you unlimited access to our entire collection of over 1,000,000 titles via our web site and mobile apps.

To claim your free month visit:

www.forgottenbooks.com/free1374913

ISBN 978-1-397-31353-9
PIBN 11374913

This book is a reproduction of an important historical work. Forgotten Books uses
state-of-the-art technology to digitally reconstruct the work, preserving the original format
whilst repairing imperfections present in the aged copy. In rare cases, an imperfection in
the original, such as a blemish or missing page, may be replicated in our edition. We do,
however, repair the vast majority of imperfections successfully; any imperfections that
remain are intentionally left to preserve the state of such historical works.

SYPHILIS

AS AFFECTING

LIFE INSURANCE RISKS

PUBLISHED BY

THE MUTUAL LIFE INSURANCE COMPANY

ON NEW YORK

1895

SYPHILIS

AS AFFECTING

LIFE INSURANCE RISKS

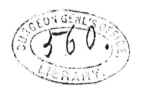

PUBLISHED BY

THE MUTUAL LIFE INSURANCE COMPANY

ON NEW YORK

1895

SYPHILIS

AS AFFECTING

LIFE INSURANCE RISKS

NEW YORK, August 7, 1895.

MR. RICHARD A. McCURDY,
President.

Sir :

I respectfully present for your consideration the following

REPORT ON SYPHILIS AS AFFECTING APPLICANTS FOR LIFE INSURANCE.

It has been hitherto the rule of The Mutual Life, under the advice of its Medical Examiners, to decline all applicants who give a history of having had syphilis. I do not know when the rule was first established, but it was probably in the early years of the Company. This rule has been enforced almost uniformly, and, if there were any exceptions, they were certainly very rare. During this long period, however, our knowledge of the natural history of this disease has been greatly increased by careful and patient observations, and there has been corresponding improvement in the methods of treatment. Consequently, the question has been raised and discussed by medical men, as to whether, with this better knowledge and treatment, the old rule might not be too rigid, and whether it should not be either annulled or at least amended, and whether such exclusion of syphilitics from the benefits of insurance was not injurious to the Company and unjust to the applicants. At the present time there is a strong preponderance of medical opinion that a syphilitic history is not to be considered an absolute bar to Life Insurance. As a matter of practice in the different Life Insurance companies the rule depends upon the personal experience, judgment or prejudice of the medical advisers. I have now endeavored to consider the question fairly and thoroughly, and to review the latest and best opinions of our medical authorities on the whole history of syphilis and its influence on the duration of the lives of those affected by it.

Syphilis begins as a local disease, arising from direct inoculation of the virus. Its first appearance is insignificant, but in a short time there is evidence of systemic infection. This is shown by certain peculiarities of the sore, glandular enlargement, fever, the appearance of characteristic spots or eruptions on the skin and mucous membrane, etc. Under appropriate treatment these manifestations may soon subside, but they are apt to recur at occasional intervals for a period of one, two, or more years, after which time they may disappear forever, leaving no sign of their former existence in the individual. In a certain percentage of cases this is the history of syphilis, even when no medical treatment has been undergone, and, with a suitable treatment, it is the history in a very large proportion.

If this were the *entire* history, there would be no question of insurance, and the disease would be regarded as only one of the minor ills of life. But, unfortunately, in a certain number of cases more grave results are observed. Occasionally in the first year, but generally after a longer period of latency, the disease shows itself in more severe and deep-seated forms, ulcerations of the skin or mucous membrane, or affections of the bones, viscera or nervous system. These local affections show no tendency to self limitation, but continue to increase or spread unless checked by medical treatment. The affections of the nervous system are the most dangerous, and at the same time, unfortunately, least amenable to treatment—some proving entirely incurable.

For while recent medical science has made progress in mitigating the severity of syphilis, it has, on the other hand, disclosed its manifestations and influence in the causation of diseases beyond what had formerly been suspected. Several serious nervous affections, as locomotor ataxia, general paralysis, and other diseases of the central nervous system, are now recognized as due to syphilis in a very large number of cases.

There is generally a period of latency between the so-called secondary symptoms and these tertiary and more severe lesions, and it is in this condition that a man will apply for insurance. The individual appears perfectly well feels perfectly well, continues well for a period varying from a few months to very many years, so that he even forgets his early sickness, and then suddenly the disease shows itself again in the form of a tumor, an ulceration, a paralysis, or other nervous affection, diseases which undoubtedly often bring life to a premature close. These eventualities must not be forgotten or glossed over in considering the question of insurance.

After this brief sketch of the natural history of syphilis, two points come up for consideration.

1. The self-limitation or curability of syphilis.

In an absolute, strict sense it can never be asserted or proved that syphilis is cured or ceases to affect an individual; and yet, in a practical common-sense view, it is often seen to be cured. If a man contracts syphilis in early life, exhibits secondary symptoms for a few years only, then lives past middle age and dies without any recurrence, in ordinary language he might reasonably be said to have been cured; but, on account of the long period of latency which is sometimes observed, the cure cannot positively be pronounced. Fournier states that he has observed tertiary syphilis first appearing fifty-five years after infection. Therefore, if our supposed case had lived a few years longer the disease might have showed itself again. Syphilitic lesions certainly reappear after a long period of apparent health, and a physician can never state positively that they will never re-appear, and pronounce his patient cured. It is in this view of the question that Gowers writes : "When we speak of the *cure* of a disease; we mean that its essential element, that which lies behind its symptoms and consequences, that which is the persistent cause behind the transient effects—we mean that this is made to cease, is ended once and for all as a morbific agent, so that it never again disturbs the system. In this sense I believe it is literally correct to say that we have no evidence that syphilis ever is or ever has been cured." Dr. Keyes expresses himself strongly to the same effect : "Hence the difficulty of saying when syphilis has ended, or indeed of deciding that it ever does end, since it so often modifies the diathesis of the individual who has suffered from it. . . . . Syphilis, once acquired, stamps its impress upon the individuality of the patient and becomes a part of him, and no power on earth in a given case can say when that impress disappears." And yet, it is the almost unanimous opinion of medical writers that the large majority of syphilitics do get well absolutely, entirely, and that it is only in a minority that these tertiary symptoms occur. Dr. Keyes writes again: "The probability of the disease in most cases, however, is that its manifestations will disappear finally after a few years, and this, under intelligent management, becomes almost a certainty." While some cases of syphilis appear to be self-limited, and come to an apparent end without having been submitted to any medical treatment, this termination or cure becomes far more probable, and it extends to a far greater proportion of cases, when an appropriate and efficient treatment has been undergone. I find that this is made by all writers an essential prerequisite before they will pronounce the probability of a patient's remaining well, and can recommend an affected individual either for marriage or for insurance.

2. In what proportion of cases of syphilis is the disease mild and of short duration, and in what proportion grave? There are no observations or statistics by which the relative numbers can be absolutely determined, and at best we can get only rough estimates made by those who have most experience in the treatment of this class of patients. These estimates range from five to twenty per cent. of severe (tertiary) cases, and it will not be far wrong to assume it as ten

per cent., that is to say, according to these authorities, that nine cases out of ten, all of which are submitted to a proper course of treatment, will remain well and free from all tertiary symptoms of the disease. One of the ten will at some subsequent period develop other and more serious lesions which may compromise his life, although most of them are still amenable to treatment. This proper course of treatment means a medical treatment and management lasting 'from one to four or more years, as may be indicated for the individual case; and, in absence of this prolonged treatment, the number and severity of tertiary cases would be far greater.

In estimating the probability of the recurrence of a disease, the lapse of time is an element of great value. It is sometimes supposed that the tertiary symptoms are apt to be late in occurring, and that after the first outburst of the disease has subsided, there will generally be a long period of latency. But, systematic observation has shown that this is not correct: while this period of latency may be very prolonged, in the majority of cases the tertiary lesions appear within a few years. Fournier gives "the following statistics based on 2,395 cases in which the date of invasion of tertiarism, under all forms of manifestation, could be determined exactly:

During the 1st year .. .. 106 cases.
During the 2d year .. .. 227 cases.
During the 3d year .. .. 256 cases.
During the 4th year .. .. 229 cases.
During the 5th year .. .. 205 cases.
During the 6th year .. .. 201 cases.

Total within 6 years 1,224
From 6th to 10th year 499
From 10th to 20th year 543
Above 20 years 129

2,395 ''

From this it appears that if the disease is to assume
the tertiary form, it will do so in more than one-half
the cases within six years, and in seventy-two per cent.
within ten years. In only twenty-eight per cent. was
the first occurrence delayed ten years.

After this brief description of the nature and course
of the disease, the original question may be considered:
Can syphilitics be insured; and, if so, under what cir-
cumstances and conditions, and how can the risk be
reduced to a minimum?

I cannot advise the abrogation of the present rule,
but only such a modification as would allow of numerous
exceptions in its practical working. The statement that
a person had had syphilis should be looked upon as an
impediment, but not as an absolute bar to life insurance.
It is an impediment that might and ought to be cleared

away by satisfactory explanation. There is a presumption of non-insurability, and the burden of proof for the removal of this presumption should rest upon the applicant.

It has been stated that the vast majority of syphilitics never have any lesions offering danger to life, provided they have taken proper treatment, but that in a small minority of cases dangerous tertiary symptoms recur. The endeavor should be to select the good and reject the bad only. I think this might be accomplished by acting according to the following suggestions:

1. No case with a history of any primary venereal sore should be accepted, until six months shall have elapsed after its first appearance. If, however, in the absence of all constitutional treatment, no other symptom, such as glandular enlargement, eruptions, mucous patches, may have appeared by this time, the applicant might be acceptable. If he has undergone any constitutional treatment, a further postponement of six months after the termination of such treatment is necessary.

2. No person with a history of syphilis is insurable, until after a proper course of treatment and the lapse of at least six years from the date of infection.

3. No person can be accepted who may have any history or evidence of tertiary manifestions.

4. On the other hand, a person may be accepted

who gives a history of constitutional syphilis, provided the original disease may not have been severe; that he shall have undergone a prolonged and satisfactory course of treatment, and a period of six years may have elapsed since the initial lesion, during the last two of which no relapses have appeared, and no tertiary symptoms at any time. I cannot advise any *rule* for the acceptance of persons who have not been submitted to proper treatment; such treatment is to be regarded not only as a great safety against future dangers, but also as an assurance that in the case of a possible re-appearance of new symptoms, medical advice would at once be sought and followed.

With regard to the time limit, I have fixed upon six years because the statistics of Fournier show that half the cases of tertiary syphilis occur during these years, and the probability of their appearances diminishes rapidly after that period. Fournier does not approve of the marriage of syphilitics until four years have elapsed, and I think that for Life Insurance six years is not too short. If the period was extended to ten years, the danger would be very considerably less. Moreover, only persons who are up to the *full* standard of physique and health should be accepted. If there is any other partial disqualification, in addition to the syphilitic history, the applicant should be declined.

As a practical matter in dealing with applications for

insurance, there is great difficulty in obtaining the information necessary to form any well grounded judgment. The answers to the printed questions are short and meagre, and often even misleading. I would recommend, therefore, that in all cases a special communication be sent to the local Examiner, with a request for such details as the Company's Medical Officers desire. This history should come, if possible, from the attending physician, but, if this be impossible, the local Examiner should certify that he is satisfied as to the accuracy of the applicant's statement. The report should give the date of the initial lesion, the kind, duration and severity of the secondary symptoms and the presence or absence of tertiary lesions, the kind and duration of the treatment, and the name of the attending physician. In want of this specific information no insurance should be approved, but, when furnished, the Company's medical adviser could generally form a correct judgment of the case. He could satisfy himself as to the *greater* or *lesser* probability of future danger, and while recognizing the impossibility of a certain prognosis, he could accept many applicants for the Company without any more risk than he assumes daily in acting upon various other classes of cases.

Respectfully,

E. J. Marsh, M. D.,
Medical Director.

November 13, 1895.

CPSIA information can be obtained
at www.ICGtesting.com
Printed in the USA
BVHW040818220219
540923BV00008B/615/P

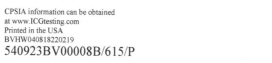